My Super Tasty Keto Diet Desserts Cookbook

Quick and Easy Delicious Desserts for Beginners and Busy people

Rebecca Marshall

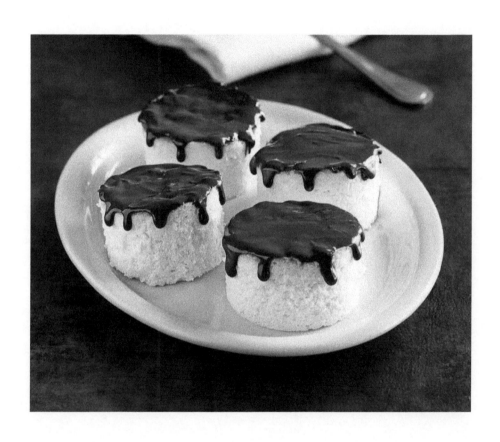

Please consult a licensed professional before attempting any techniques outlined in this book.

By reading this document, the reader agrees that under no circumstances is the author responsible for any losses, direct or indirect, which are incurred as a result of the use of information contained within this document, including, but not limited to, — errors, omissions, or inaccuracies.

Table of contents

Apple Cinnamon Chaffles

Preparation Time: 5 minutes

Cooking Time: 4 minutes

Serving: 3

Ingredients:

- Eggs (3)
- Shredded mozzarella cheese (1 cup)
- Chopped apple (.25 cup)
- Monk fruit sweetener (.5 tsp.)
- Gluten-free baking powder (.25 tsp.)
- Coconut flour (2 tbsp.)
- Cinnamon (1.5 tsp.)

Directions:

1. Warm the Chaffle maker while you whisk the eggs until they are frothy.
2. Mix them with the rest of the fixings and pour 1/3 of the batter at a time into the heated cooked. Cooking them until golden brown (4 min.). Serve when all are prepared.

Nutrition:

Calories: 101

Net Carb: 1.6g

Fat: 7.1g

Carbohydrates: 2.9g

Dietary Fiber: 1.3g

Banana Nut Chaffles

Preparation Time: 5 minutes

Cooking Time: 4 minutes

Serving: 3

Ingredients:

- Egg (1)
- Unchilled cream cheese - softened (1 tbsp.)
- Optional: Sugar-free cheesecake pudding (1 tbsp. - Note: The mix is 'dirty' keto)
- Mozzarella cheese (.5 cup)
- Monk fruit confectioners (1 tbsp.)
- Vanilla extracts (.25 tsp.)
- Banana extracts (.25 tsp.)

Optional Toppings:

- Sugar-free caramel sauce
- Pecans/any of your favorite nuts

Directions:

1. Preheat the mini Chaffle maker. In a small bowl, merge the egg and add the remaining ingredients to the egg mixture, mixing until it's well incorporated. Add half the batter to the Chaffle maker and Cooking it for a minimum of four minutes until its golden brown.
2. Remove the finished chaffle and add the other half of the batter to Cooking the other chaffle. Top with your optional ingredients and serve warm.

Nutrition:

Cal 468

Net Carbs 2g

Fat 38g

Protein 26g

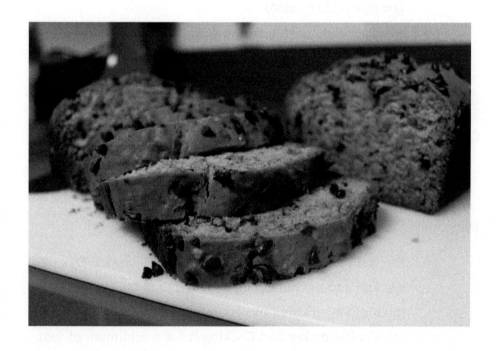

Brownie Chaffle - Keto

Preparation Time: 5 minutes

Cooking Time: 4 minutes

Serving: 3

Ingredients:

- Egg (1)
- Shredded mozzarella cheese (.33 cup)
- Cocoa powder - Dutch-processed/regular (1.5 tbsp.)
- Almond flour (1 tbsp.)
- Monk fruit Sweetener (1 tbsp. + 1 tsp. if you like your treats sweeter)
- Vanilla extracts (.25 tsp.)
- Baking powder (.25 tsp.)
- Salt (1 pinch)
- Optional: Heavy cream (2 tsp.)

Directions:

1. Preheat a mini-Chaffle iron. Whisk the egg and add the dry ingredients. Add the cheese. Note: If you want a moist chaffle, add two tablespoons of heavy cream to the batter.
2. Pour 1/3 of the batter on the Chaffle iron. Cooking for three minutes or until steam stops coming out of the Chaffle iron. Slightly cool on a wire rack. Serve with your favorite low-carb toppings.

Nutrition:

Cal 263

Net Carbs: 6g

Fat: 22g

Protein: 10g

Cherry Chocolate Chaffle

Preparation Time: 5 minutes

Cooking Time: 15 minutes

Serving: 1

Ingredients:

- Unsweetened chocolate chips (1 tbsp.)
- Lightly beaten egg (1)
- Sugar-free cherry pie filling (2 tbsp.)
- Heavy whipping cream (2 tbsp.)
- Shredded mozzarella cheese (.5 cup)
- Gluten-free baking powder (.5 tsp.)
- Unsweetened cocoa powder (1 tbsp.)
- Swerve (1 tbsp.)
- Almond flour (1 tbsp.)

Directions:

1. Preheat the Chaffle iron and spray using Cooking oil spray. Whisk the flour, cocoa powder, Swerve, baking powder, cheese, and egg. Empty the batter into the hot Chaffle maker and Cooking until it's golden like you like them.
2. Garnish them with the pie filling, whipping cream and chocolate chips to serve.

Nutrition:

Cal 89

Net Carbs 5.9g

Fat 6g

Protein 2g

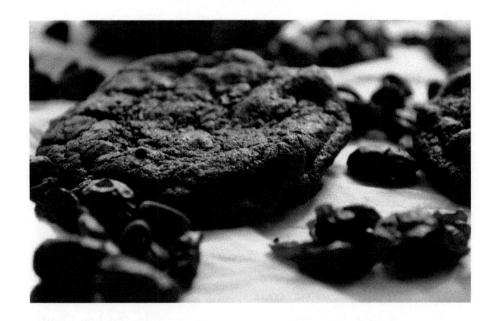

Choco Chip Lemon Chaffle

Preparation Time: 5 minutes

Cooking Time: 15 minutes

Serving: 1

Ingredients:

- Unsweetened chocolate chips (1 tbsp.)
- Lightly whisked eggs (2)
- Vanilla (.5 tsp.)
- Swerve (2 tsp.)
- Lemon extracts (.5 tsp.)
- Shredded mozzarella (.5 cup)
- Almond flour (2 tsp.)

Directions:

1. Warm the Chaffle maker and spritz the grids with a non-stick Cooking oil spray. Whisk each of the fixings in a mixing bowl and pour half of it into the Chaffle iron.
2. Cooking for four to five minutes. Transfer to a platter and Cooking the second chaffle. Serve when both are ready as desired.

Nutrition:

Cal 151

Net Carbs: 2g

Fat: 11g

Protein: 7g

Choco and Strawberry Chaffle

Preparation Time: 5 minutes

Cooking Time: 20 minutes

Serving: 2

Ingredients:

- Strawberry puree (.5 cup)
- Almond flour (1 tbsp.)
- Cocoa powder (1 tbsp.)
- Baking powder (.5 tsp.)
- Cheddar cheese (.5 cup)
- Large egg (1)
- Optional: Vanilla extracts (.5 tsp.)
- Melted coconut oil (2 tbsp.)

Directions:

1. Warm the mini Chaffle maker and lightly spritz the grids using a Cooking spray. Melt the oil in a microwave. Whisk the baking powder and flour. Whisk the egg, oil, cheese puree, and oil with the dry fixings. Dust the iron using about 1/8 cup of cheese.
2. Mix the batter thoroughly and pour in the batter in batches to make the chaffle. Sprinkle with more cheese and securely close the lid. Prepare them for four to five minutes until they are crispy as desired.

Nutrition:

Cal 209

Net Carbs 2.7g;

Fat 17g

Protein 8g

Simple Chocolate Chaffle

Preparation Time: 5 minutes

Cooking Time: 20 minutes

Serving: 1

Ingredients:

- Lightly whisked egg (1)
- Monk fruit (1.5 tsp.)
- Vanilla (1 tsp.)
- Unsweetened cocoa powder (1 tbsp.)
- Cream cheese (1 oz.)
- Almond flour (2 tbsp.)

Directions:

1. Warm the Chaffle iron and spritz the grids using Cooking oil spray. Whisk the egg, monk fruit, vanilla, cream cheese, almond flour, and cocoa powder. Empty the batter into the hot Chaffle iron using two batches.
2. Serve when they are crispy to your liking.

Nutrition:

Calories: 122

Net Carb: 0.5g

Fat: 9.4g

Carbohydrates: 0.5g

Chocolate Twinkle Chaffle

Preparation Time: 15 minutes

Cooking Time: 25 minutes

Serving: 6

Ingredients:

- Butter - melted and cooled (2 tbsp.)
- Cream cheese (2 oz. - softened)
- Unchilled eggs (2 large)
- Vanillas extract (1 tsp.)
- Lakanto Confectioners (.25 cup)
- Pink salt (1 pinch)
- Almond flour (.25 cup)
- Baking powder (1 tsp.)
- Coconut flour (2 tbsp.)
- Cacao powder (2 tbsp.)

Directions:

1. Preheat the Corn Dog Maker. Melt the butter and let it cool for minute. Whisk the eggs into the butter until creamy. Whisk in the sweetener, vanilla, and salt. Mix the almond flour, coconut flour, cacao powder, and baking powder until well incorporated.

2. Add two tablespoons of batter to each well and spread across evenly. Close the lid, lock, and Cooking it for four minutes. Remove and cool them on a rack.

Nutrition:

Calories: 56

Net Carb: 0.4g

Fat: 3.7g

Carbohydrates: 0.4g

Dietary Fiber: 0g

Keto Cinnamon Cream Cheese Chaffle

Preparation Time: 15 minutes

Cooking Time: 25 minutes

Serving: 2

Ingredients:

- Lightly whisked eggs (2)
- Collagen (1 tsp.)
- Monk fruit sweetener (1 tsp.)
- Gluten-free baking powder (.25 tsp.)
- Unchilled cream cheese (.25 cup)
- Salt (1 pinch)
- Cinnamon (.5 tsp.)

Directions:

1. Warm the mini Chaffle iron while you combine all of the fixings.
2. Spray the heated grids using a spritz of Cooking oil spray. Whisk half of the batter into the Chaffle maker and Cooking for three to four minutes until they're golden to your liking.

Nutrition:

Cal 467

Net Carbs 3.2g;

Fat 37g

Protein 27g

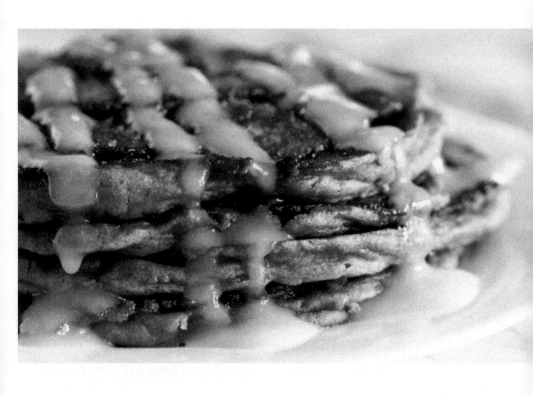

Cinnamon Roll Swirl Chaffle

Preparation Time: 15 minutes

Cooking Time: 30 minutes

Serving: 3

Ingredients:

Chaffle Ingredients:

- Mozzarella cheese (.5 cup)
- Almond flour (1 tbsp.)
- Baking powder (.25 tsp.)
- Eggs (1)
- Cinnamon (1 tsp.)
- Granulated Swerve (1 tsp.)

Cinnamon Roll Swirl Ingredients:

- Butter (1 tbsp.)
- Cinnamon (1 tsp.)
- Confectioners swerve (2 tsp.)

Keto Cinnamon Roll Glaze:

- Butter (1 tbsp.)
- Cream cheese (1 tbsp.)
- Vanilla extracts (.25 tsp.)
- Swerve confectioners (2 tsp.)

Directions:

1. Start the mini Chaffle maker to heat. Whisk the chaffle ingredients and set it to the side for now. Use another

container and add the swirl ingredients. Microwave it for 15 seconds, mixing well. Use a non-stick Cooking oil spray to prepare the Chaffle iron. Swirl the cinnamon, swerve, and butter mixture. Pour (1 /3 of the batter) and add it over the chaffle fixings.

2. Close the Chaffle maker and Cooking for three to four minutes. Continue the process until the batter is used, and you have three chaffle. While the third chaffle is Cooking, place one tablespoon of butter and one tablespoon of cream cheese in a bowl. Heat it for 10 seconds. If the cream cheese still is not softened, set it for another 5 seconds. Stir in the swerve confectioners sweetener and vanilla extract. Whisk and drizzle the glaze over the chaffle and serve.

Nutrition:

Calories: 145

Net Carb: 0.5g

Fat: 11.6g

Carbohydrates: 0.5g

Dietary Fiber: 0g

Cocoa Chaffle

Preparation Time: 15 minutes

Cooking Time: 30 minutes

Serving: 2

Ingredients:

- Shredded cheddar cheese (.5 cup)
- Large egg (1)
- Almond flour (2 tbsp.)
- Cocoa powder (1 tbsp.)

Directions:

1. Heat the Chaffle maker using the med-high temperature setting. Whisk the ingredients in a mixing bowl. Prepare it in two batches.
2. Add the batter to the cooker and prepare it for three to five minutes. After the second chaffle is browned, serve them hot.

Nutrition:

Cal 215

Net Carbs 4g

Fat 15g

Protein 12g

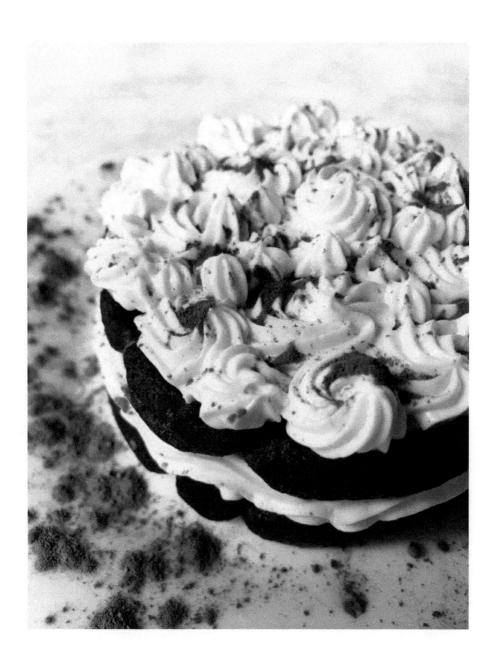

Deluxe Cocoa Chaffle With Coconut Cream

Preparation Time: 5 minutes

Cooking Time: 20 minutes

Serving: 2

Ingredients:

- Mozzarella cheese (.5 cup)
- Egg (1)
- Vanilla (1 tsp.)
- Stevia (1 tsp.)
- Almond flour (2 tbsp.)
- Cocoa powder (2 tbsp.)
- Sugar-free chocolate chips (1 tbsp.)

The Topping:

- Coconut cream (1 scoop)
- Coconut flour (1 tbsp.)

Directions:

1. Combine and whisk the chaffle fixings. Warm the mini Chaffle maker and spritz it using a bit of Cooking oil spray. prepare the two servings in batches (4 chaffle) and pour the batter into the Chaffle iron.
2. Cooking each batch for two to four minutes or until they are crispy. Serve with a scoop of the coconut cream between

two of the chaffle. Finish it off using a dusting of coconut flour and serve.

Nutrition:

Cal 89

Net Carbs 5.9g

Fat 6g

Protein 2g

Gingerbread Chaffle

Preparation Time: 5 minutes

Cooking Time: 20 minutes

Serving: 2

Ingredients:

- Grated mozzarella cheese (.5 cup)
- Egg (1 medium)
- Baking powder (.5 tsp.)
- Powdered Erythritol (1 tsp.)
- Ground ginger (.5 tsp.)
- Almond flour (2 tbsp.)
- Ground cloves (.125 tsp.)
- Cinnamon (.5 tsp.)
- Nutmeg (.25 tsp.)

Directions:

1. Turn on the Chaffle maker and lightly grease it with a bit of olive oil. Whisk the egg and add the rest of the fixings. Add the batter in two batches and Cooking for about five minutes.
2. Remove the chaffle using tongs and serve with cream cheese frosting or whipped cream.

Nutrition:

Cal 215

Net Carbs 4g

Fat 15g

Protein 12g

Maple Chaffle

Preparation Time: 5 minutes

Cooking Time: 20 minutes

Serving: 2

Ingredients:

- Egg whites (2)
- Whole egg (1)
- Maple extracts (.5 tsp.)
- Swerve (2 tsp.)
- GF baking powder (.5 tsp.)
- Almond milk (2 tbsp.
- Coconut flour (2 tbsp.)

Directions:

1. Before Preparation, warm the mini Chaffle maker. Set the egg whites and form stiff peaks. Stir in the rest of the fixings. Spray the Chaffle maker with a nonstick Cooking spray. Pour half of the batter after its heated, and Cooking for three to five minutes.
2. Pour in the last of the batter and Cooking the same time before serving.

Nutrition:

Calories: 147

Net Carb: 1.2g

Fat: 11.5g

Carbohydrates: 1.2g

Dietary Fiber: 0g

Mint Chocolate Brownie Chaffle

Preparation Time: 5 minutes

Cooking Time: 20 minutes

Serving: 12

Ingredients:

The Base:

- Butter (.5 cup)
- Chocolate chips - Sugar-free (1 cup)
- Superfine almond flour (1 cup)

The Topping:

- Butter - softened (.25 cup)
- Powdered Swerve (.33 cup)
- Heavy whipping cream (6 tbsp.)
- Peppermint extracts (1 tsp.)
- Optional: Green food coloring (1 drop)
- Also Needed: 8 x 6-inch square pan

Directions:

1. Lightly grease the pan with a spritz of Cooking oil or spray. Toss the chocolate and butter in a microwave-safe bowl. Heat the mixture for 15-20 seconds in the microwave, stirring until it is all melted. Add in the almond flour and mix well. Pat this mixture into the prepared pan and place it in the fridge. Beat the whipping cream, 1/4 cup butter, peppermint extract, and food color with an electric mixer

using the medium speed setting until it's well mixed. Using the low-speed setting gradually beat in powdered Swerve until smooth. Spread the peppermint mixture evenly over chocolate mixture. Refrigerate for 15 to 20 minutes.

2. Slice the chilled mix into five rows by five rows. Be careful not to over-microwave the chocolate or start to harden and ruin the recipe. The best practice is to stir to allow the melted butter to melt the chocolate the rest of the way.

Nutrition:

Cal 199

Net Carbs 4.7g

Fat 20g

Protein 3g

Peanut Butter Chaffle

Preparation Time: 5 minutes

Cooking Time: 20 minutes

Serving: 2

Ingredients:

- Creamy peanut butter - keto-friendly (2 tbsp.)
- Shredded mozzarella cheese (.25 cup)
- Almond flour (1 tbsp.)
- Egg (1)
- Unsweetened chocolate chips (1 tbsp.)
- Vanilla (.5 tsp.)
- Swerve (1 tbsp.)

Directions:

1. Heat the mini Chaffle iron. Spritz the grids using a Cooking spray. Whisk the egg and peanut butter in a mixing container. Fold in the chips, cheese, flour, and swerve.
2. Prepare the chaffle in two batches, Cooking for about four minutes each, and serve.

Nutrition:

Calories: 101

Net Carb: 1.6g

Fat: 7.1g

Carbohydrates: 2.9g

Dietary Fiber: 1.3g

Peanut Butter Brownie Chaffle

Preparation Time: 5 minutes

Cooking Time: 15 minutes

Serving: 2

Ingredients:

- Shredded mozzarella cheese (.5 cup)
- Cocoa powder (1 tbsp.)
- Powdered sweetener - ex. Swerve Confectioners (2 tbsp.)
- Peanut butter - Sugar-free (2 tbsp.)
- Vanilla (.5 tsp.)
- Egg (1)

Optional For the Topping 2 tbsp. of each:

- Crushed peanuts
- Whipped cream

Directions:

1. Mix the egg, shredded mozzarella, peanut butter, vanilla, sweetener, and cocoa powder in a mixing bowl. Fold in the peanuts, if desired, and arrange them on a plate. Warm the Chaffle maker and spritz with some Cooking oil. Set half of the batter into the Chaffle iron and close the lid. Cooking for four minutes before arranging on a plate.
2. Top each one off using whipped cream and more nuts or sugar- free chips before serving.

Nutrition:

Cal 239

Net Carbs 3g

Fat 15g

Protein 9g

Pecan Pumpkin Chaffle

Preparation Time: 5 minutes

Cooking Time: 20 minutes

Serving: 2

Ingredients:

- Eggs (1)
- Erythritol (1 tsp.)
- Almond flour (2 tbsp.)
- Toasted and chopped pecans (2 tbsp.)
- Pumpkin purees (1 tbsp.)
- Pumpkin pie spice (.25 tsp.)
- Grated mozzarella cheese.

Directions:

1. Plug in the Chaffle maker to preheat. Spray the grids with a non- stick baking spray. Whisk the egg and add the remainder of the fixings to prepare the batter.
2. Pour the batter into the Chaffle iron using two batches. Cooking them for five minutes until they are crispy and serve.

Nutrition:

Calories 235

Fats 20.62g

Carbs 5.9g

Net Carbs 5g

Protein 7.51g

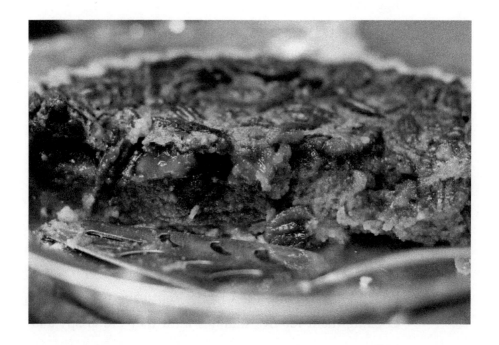

Pumpkin Chaffle with Frosting

Preparation Time: 15 minutes

Cooking Time: 25 minutes

Serving: 2

Ingredients:

- Egg (1 beaten)
- Sugar-free pumpkin puree (1 tbsp.)
- Shredded mozzarella cheese (.5 cup)
- Pumpkin pie spice (.25 tsp.)

The Frosting:

- Swerve (2 tbsp.)
- Vanilla (.5 tsp.)
- Unchilled cream cheese (2 tbsp.)

Directions:

1. Warm the Chaffle maker and spray it using a nonstick baking spray. Whisk the chaffle fixings and pour half of the batter into the mini cooker to Cook for three to four minutes.
2. Make the second chaffle. Prepare the frosting fixings and spread it over the chaffle to serve.

Nutrition:

Calories 210

Total Fat 17 g

Saturated Fat 10 g

Cholesterol 110 mg

Sodium 250 mg

Potassium 570 mg

Easy Pumpkin Cheesecake Chaffle

Preparation Time: 5 minutes

Cooking Time: 20 minutes

Serving: 2

Ingredients:

The chaffle:

- Vanilla (.5 tsp.)
- Egg (1)
- Gluten-free baking powder (.5 tsp.)
- Unchilled cream cheese (1 tsp.)
- Pumpkin spice (.25 tsp.)
- Heavy cream (2 tsp.)
- Swerve (1 tbsp.)
- Almond flour (1 tbsp.)
- Shredded mozzarella cheese (.5 cup)
- Pumpkin puree (2 tsp.)

For the Filling:

- Cream cheese (2 tbsp.)
- Swerve (1 tbsp.)
- Vanilla (.25 tsp.)

Directions:

1. Warm the mini Chaffle iron and spritz it with a Cooking oil spray. Whisk each of the chaffle fixings and pour half of the batter into the heated maker.

2. Cooking it for three to five minutes, and Cooking the second one. Mix the filling ingredients in a mixing bowl and spread between the Prepare chaffle. Pop them into the fridge for about ten minutes before serving.

Nutrition:

Cal 112

Net Carbs 4g

Fat 5g

Protein 9g

Belgium Chaffle

Preparation Time: 5 minutes

Cooking Time: 6 minutes

Serving: 1

Ingredients:

- 1 cup grated cheddar cheese
- 2 eggs

Directions:

1. Preheat the Chaffle iron.
2. Beat the eggs then add the grated cheddar cheese.
3. Make sure that the mixture is well combined.
4. Cooking the mixture for about six minutes.

Nutrition

Calories: 460

Cholesterol: 490 mg

Carbohydrates: 2 g

Protein: 44 g

Fat: 33 g

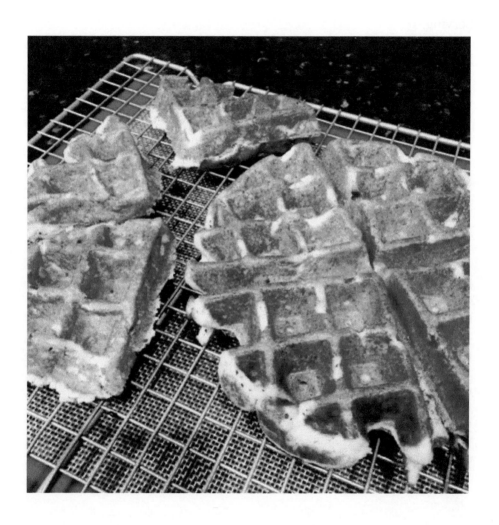

Apple Pie Chaffle

Preparation Time: 45 minutes

Cooking Time: 15 minutes

Serving: 8

Ingredients:

Chaffle Ingredients:

- 3 eggs
- 1 1/2 cups grated cheddar cheese

Ingredients for Toppings:

- 4 Gala apples (1 1/4 lb.), chopped finely
- 1/2 tsp. ground cinnamon
- 1/4 cup sugar
- 2 tbsp. butter, melted
- 1/4 cup pecans, chopped
- 1/2 cup whipped cream

Directions:

Chaffle

1. Preheat the Chaffle iron.
2. Combine the eggs and cheese well.
3. Roughly 2 tbsp. is 1 mini chaffle.
4. Attach the batter to the Chaffle iron and Cooking for about three minutes.
5. A total of eight chaffles can be made with this batter.
6. Allow to cool and start on the topping.

Directions

Topping:

1. Take the butter and melt in the saucepan at medium heat.
2. Add the chopped apples and Cooking for two minutes stirring often.
3. Attach the cinnamon and sugar to the apples.
4. Mix the pecans into the mixture and stir in.
5. Cover the saucepan with a lid and Cooking for a further five minutes at a low temperature.
6. Apples should be cooked until tender.

Nutrition

Calories: 250 kcal

Cholesterol: 100 mg

Carbohydrates: 21 g

Protein: 8 g

Fat: 16 g

Sugar: 16 g

French toast Chaffle

Preparation Time: 5 minutes

Cooking Time: 10 minutes

Serving: 2

Ingredients:

- 1 egg
- 1/2 cup grated mozzarella cheese
- 2 tbsp. almond flour,
- 1 tsp. vanilla extract
- 1 tsp. cinnamon
- 1 tsp. granulated sweetener of choice

Directions:

1. Preheat your Chaffle iron.
2. Mix all the chaffle ingredients well.
3. Use half of the mixture and Cooking the chaffle for about five minutes.
4. Add an extra minute to the Cooking if you want a crispier chaffle.
5. Repeat until all the batter is used.
6. Add some sugar-free cinnamon syrup and enjoy these chaffles still warm.

Nutrition

Calories: 180 kcal

Carbohydrates: 7 g

Protein: 11 g

Fat: 12 g

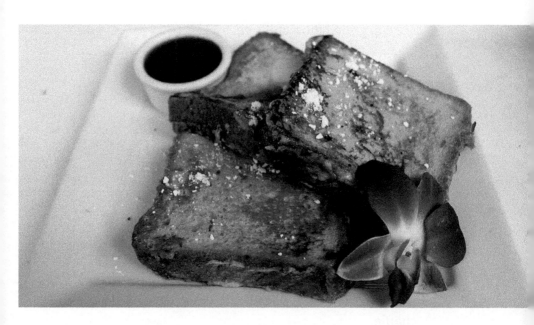

Banana Nut Chaffle Recipe

Preparation Time: 3 minutes

Cooking Time: 8 minutes

Serving: 2

Ingredients:

- 1 egg
- 1/4 tsp. vanilla extract
- 1/4 tsp. banana extract
- 1 tbsp. cream cheese, room temperature, and softened
- 1/2 cup grated mozzarella cheese
- 1 tbsp. monk fruit confectioners, or confectioners sweetener of choice
- 1 tbsp. sugar-free cheesecake pudding, optional

Toppings:

- Pecans
- Sugar-free caramel sauce. or keto-safe sauce of preference

Directions:

1. Preheat the Chaffle iron.
2. Set the egg before adding the other ingredients and make sure that everything is coated in the egg mixture.
3. Use half of the batter and Cooking for about four minutes.
4. Remove chaffle to rest while Cooking the second mini chaffle.

Nutrition

Calories: 119 kcal

Cholesterol: 111 mg

Carbohydrates: 2.7 g

Protein: 8.8 g

Fat: 7.8 g

Sugar: 1.1 g

Banana Foster Chaffle Pancakes

Preparation Time: 3 minutes

Cooking Time: 20 minutes

Serving: 4

Ingredients:

Chaffle Ingredients:

- 4 large eggs
- 1 cup almond flour, ALLERGY WARNING
- 1/3 cup flaxseed meal
- 1 tsp. vanilla extract
- 1/2 medium banana, slightly overripe
- 4 oz. cream cheese
- 2 tsp. baking powder
- 1/2 tsp. banana extract, optional
- Liquid stevia or sweetener of choice, optional

Ingredients for Banana Foster Topping:

- 8 tbsp. salted butter
- 1/2 tsp. cinnamon
- 1/2 tsp. vanilla extract
- 1/2 tsp. banana extract
- 1/4 cup sugar-free maple syrup
- 1/2 cup brown sugar substitute or granulated sweetener with maple extract
- 1/2 medium banana, sliced into discs

- 1/8-1/4 tsp. xanthan gum, optional
- 2 tbsp. dark rum or bourbon, optional
- 1/4 cup pecans chopped, optional

Directions:

1. Preheat the Chaffle iron or skillet.
2. Add all the chaffle ingredients to a blender and blend until smooth.
3. Add 1/4 of the batter to the Chaffle iron and Cooking for about two–three minutes, add an extra minute to Cooking if the chaffle isn't set.
4. Repeat until all the batter is used.

Directions of Topping:

1. At a medium temperature combine the banana extract, rum or bourbon, butter, and vanilla in a skillet.
2. As the mixture starts to bubble, attach the sliced bananas in a single layer and allow them to Cooking for between two to three minutes. Do not stir.
3. After the time has passed, add the cinnamon, brown sugar substitute, and sugar-free maple syrup.
4. Stir and let the mixture simmer until all the brown sugar substitute has become melted and incorporated into the butter.
5. If the brown sugar substitute isn't blending with the butter, then add the xanthan gum to the simmering mixture. This will also help to thicken up the sauce.

6. Depending on your preference, you can either add the pecans to the simmering sauce or add it after pouring the source on the chaffles.

7. Add the warm sauce to the cooled chaffles.

8. Add a scoop or two of keto-friendly ice cream to make a unique taste experience. Or simply enjoy the chaffle with no sauce.

Nutrition

Calories: 417 kcal

Cholesterol: 170 mg

Carbohydrates: 13 g

Protein: 10 g

Fat: 37 g

Sugar: 7 g

Chocolate Chip Chaffles

Preparation Time: 3 minutes

Cooking Time: 8 minutes

Serving: 2

Ingredients:

- 1/2 cup grated mozzarella cheese
- 1/2 tbsp. granulated Swerve, or sweetener of choice
- 1 tbsp. almond flour, ALLERGY WARNING
- 2 tbsp. low carb, sugar-free chocolate chips
- 1 egg
- 1/4 tsp. cinnamon

Directions:

1. Preheat your Chaffle iron.
2. In a bowl, merge the almond flour, egg, cinnamon, mozzarella cheese, Swerve, chocolate chips.
3. Place half the batter in the Chaffle iron and Cooking for four minutes.
4. Remove chaffle and Cooking the remaining batter.
5. Let chaffles cool before serving.

Nutrition

Calories: 136 kcal

Cholesterol: 104 mg

Carbohydrates: 2 g

Protein: 10 g

Fat: 10 g

Sugar: 1 g

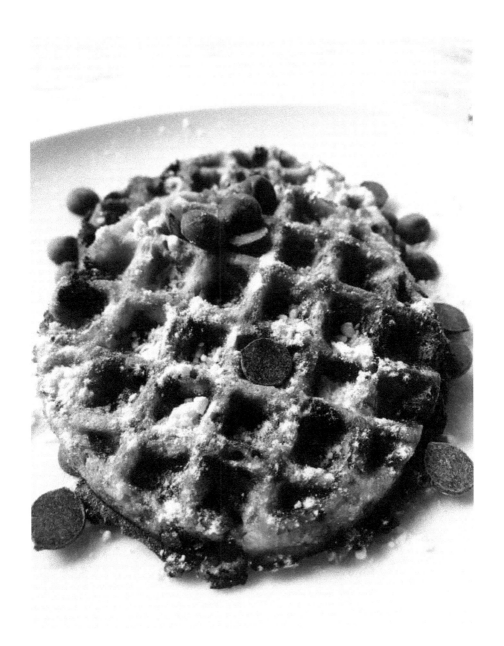

Chocolate Chaffle Recipe

Preparation Time: 3 minutes

Cooking Time: 8 minutes

Serving: 2

Ingredients:

- 1 tsp. vanilla extract
- 1 tbsp. cocoa powder, unsweetened.
- 1 egg
- 2 tbsp. almond flour, ALLERGY WARNING
- 2 tsp. monk fruit
- 1 oz. cream cheese

Directions:

1. Preheat the Chaffle iron.
2. Soften the cream cheese then whisk together the other ingredients well.
3. Set the batter into the center of the Chaffle iron and spread out.
4. Cooking batter for between three and five minutes.
5. Remove chaffle once set and serve.

Nutrition

Calories: 261 kcal

Carbohydrates: 4 g net

Protein: 11.5 g

Fat: 22.2 g

S'mores Chaffles

Preparation Time: 30 minutes

Cooking Time: 20 minutes

Serving: 2

Ingredients:

Chaffle Ingredients:

- 1 egg
- 1/2 tsp. vanilla extract
- 1/4 cup cream cheese
- 2 tbsp. almond flour, ALLERGY WARNING
- 1 tbsp. sweetener of choice
- 1 tbsp. protein powder, unflavored
- 1/2 tsp. baking powder
- 1 tsp. ground cinnamon

For Sugar-Free Marshmallow:

- 100 g (3.5 oz.,) xylitol, or other baking friendly sweetener
- 3 tbsp. water
- 4 gelatin sheets, or 7 g gelatin powder

For Chocolate Dip:

- 10 g cacao butter
- 80 g sugar-free chocolate

Directions for Sugar-Free Marshmallow:

1. If you do not have sugar-free marshmallow fluff, then it is suggested that you make this up to eight hours, or even the day before, making the chaffle.
2. Choose a container to set the marshmallow in later. This container needs to be lined with cling film.
3. Gelatin sheets need to be placed in water for a few minutes before use.
4. Melt the sugar in a Cooking pot and allow boiling for up to three minutes before adding the gelatin sheets or powder.
5. Dissolve the gelatin fully.
6. Now that the liquid is ready, pour it into an electric mixer.
7. Mix the mixture until the liquid bulks up and starts to form a white marshmallow-like fluff.
8. Pour the marshmallow fluff into the previously prepared container and smooth the surface.
9. Allow the mixture to sit on a kitchen surface for no less than eight hours. For the best possible setting, allow for the fluff to rest overnight to allow it to set into the marshmallow form. Cover with cling film once cool to prevent insects from getting into the mixture.
10. Once fully set, the marshmallow can be cut into the desired shape.
11. Dust the marshmallow pieces with powdered sweetener if you want to keep it softer for longer.

Chaffle Directions:

1. Preheat the Chaffle iron.
2. Beat the egg before adding the cinnamon.

3. Combine the remaining chaffle ingredients before adding a few drops of vanilla.
4. Divide the batter in half and Cooking each portion for three minutes.
5. Set chaffles aside to cool.
6. If you want to prepare the s'mores at home, take the marshmallow fluff and spread it to the thickness of choice on one chaffle before adding the second chaffle on top.
7. Set aside the chaffles to prepare the chocolate dip.

Directions for Chocolate Dip:

1. Make use of a double boiler or instant pot to melt the cocoa butter and sugar-free chocolate together.
2. Make sure the mixture is completely smooth before dipping the chaffle's edges in it. Coat all the marshmallow fluff.
3. Put aside and allow the chocolate to harden.

Nutrition

Calories: 368 kcal

Carbohydrates: 3 g

Protein: 11 g

Fat: 23 g

Thin Mint Cookies Chaffles

Preparation Time: 20 minutes

Cooking Time: 16 minutes

Serving: 4

Ingredients:

Chaffle Ingredients:

- 1 cup grated mozzarella cheese
- 2 tbsp. unsweetened cocoa powder
- 2 large eggs
- 3 tbsp. Swerve confectioners, or sweetener of choice

For Filling:

- 6 oz. cream cheese, softened
- 2 tbsp. unsweetened cocoa powder
- 1/2 cup almond flour
- 1/4 cup Swerve confectioners, or sweeteners of choice
- 1 tsp. peppermint extract
- 1/2 tsp. vanilla extract

For Topping:

- 3 tbsp. sugar-free chocolate chips
- 1 tbsp. coconut oil, ALLERGY WARNING

Directions:

For Chaffle

1. Preheat the Chaffle iron.

2. Mix all the chaffle ingredients in a bowl and make sure everything is mixed well.

3. Cooking 1/4 of the batter in the Chaffle iron for two to four minutes. The longer it is cooked, the crispier it becomes.

4. Continue to make chaffles until the batter is finished.

Directions

For Filling and Topping:

1. Combine all the filler ingredients and beat with a hand mixer on high.

2. Apply the filling to the three cooled chaffles, stack, and set aside.

3. Heat the coconut oil and chocolate chips at 30-second intervals in a microwave until melted together.

4. Drizzle this over the stacked chaffles and serve.

Nutrition

Calories: 431 kcal

Carbohydrates: 6 g net

Protein: 16 g

Fat: 38 g

Strawberry Chaffle

Preparation Time: 20 minutes

Cooking Time: 16 minutes

Serving: 2

Ingredients:

- Sliced strawberries (2 fresh)
- Egg (1)
- Vanilla (1 tsp.)
- Baking powder (.25 tsp.)
- Shredded mozzarella cheese (.25 cup)
- Cream cheese (1 tbsp.)

Directions:

1. Preheat the mini Chaffle maker and spritz with a bit of Cooking spray. Whisk the egg and add the rest of the fixings to make the batter.
2. Prepare the batter in two batches, Cooking them until golden or about four minutes.

Nutrition:

Calories 210

Total Fat 17 g

Saturated Fat 10 g

Cholesterol 110 mg

Sodium 250 mg

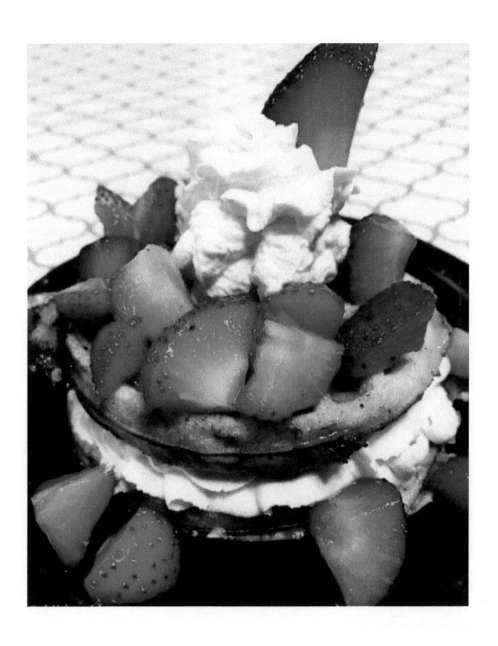

Chocolate Ice Cream Sundae Chaffle

Preparation Time: 5 minutes

Cooking Time: 20 minutes

Serving: 3

Ingredients:

Ingredients:

- 1 egg
- 1/2 tsp. baking powder
- 1 tsp. vanilla extract
- 1/2 cup grated mozzarella cheese
- 2 tbsp. unsweetened cocoa powder
- 3 tbsp. Swerve sweetener, or sweetener of choice

Toppings:

- 2 cups keto-friendly vanilla ice cream
- Pecans
- Keto-friendly chocolate sauce

Directions:

1. Preheat the Chaffle iron.
2. Mix all the ingredients well.
3. Use 1/3 of the batter to make a mini chaffle and Cooking for between five to seven minutes.
4. Allow each cooked chaffle to cool completely.

Nutrition

Calories: 128 kcal

Cholesterol: 104 mg

Carbohydrates: 3 g

Protein: 9.5 g

Fat: 8.7 g

Sugar: 0.7 g

Fudgy Chocolate Dessert Chaffles

Preparation Time: 5 minutes

Cooking Time: 20 minutes

Serving: 4

Ingredients:

- 2 large eggs
- 2 tsp. coconut flour, ALLERGY WARNING
- 4 tbsp. grated mozzarella cheese
- 2 tbsp. heavy whipping cream
- 1/2 tsp. baking powder
- 1/2 tsp. vanilla extract
- 1 tbsp. dark cacao (70 percent cocoa or higher)
- Pinch of salt
- 1/4 tsp. Stevia powder, or powdered sweetener of choice

Directions:

1. Preheat the Chaffle iron.
2. Beat the eggs and cream together before adding the other ingredients to the mixture.
3. Divide the batter into four parts and add to the Chaffle iron.
4. Cooking the chaffles for about three to five minutes then remove them from the Chaffle iron.
5. Continue until all the batter is gone.

Nutrition

Calories: 83 kcal

Cholesterol: 102.7 mg

Carbohydrates: 3 g

Protein: 6.1 g

Fat: 5.4 g

Sugar: 0.8 g

Pumpkin Pecan Chaffle

Preparation Time: 2 minutes

Cooking Time: 10 minutes

Serving: 2

Ingredients:

- 1 egg
- 2 tbsp. almond flour, ALLERGY WARNING
- 2 tbsp. pecans, toasted chopped
- 1/2 cup mozzarella cheese grated
- 1/2 tsp. pumpkin spice
- 1 tbsp. pumpkin puree, sugar-free
- 1 tsp. Erythritol low carb, or sweetener of choice

Directions:

1. Preheat the Chaffle iron.
2. First, beat the egg before adding the other ingredients. Make sure everything is coated by the egg.
3. Depending on the size of your Chaffle iron spoon in the necessary amount. Don't overfill.
4. Cooking the batter for about five minutes and repeat with the remaining batter if there is.

Nutrition

Calories: 210 kcal

Carbohydrates: 4.6 g

Protein: 11 g

Fat: 17 g

Maple Pecan Chaffles

Preparation Time: 5 minutes

Cooking Time: 8 minutes

Serving: 2

Ingredients:

- 1 large egg
- 1 tbsp. sweetener of choice
- 2-3 drops maple flavoring
- 1/2 cup grated mozzarella cheese
- 1 tbsp. pecans, chopped
- 1/4 cup almond flour,

Directions:

1. Preheat the Chaffle iron.
2. Whisk eggs before adding the chopped pecans, sweetener, maple flavoring, mozzarella cheese, almond flour. Mix well.
3. Take half the batter and Cooking for between three to four minutes.
4. Repeat until the batter is used up completely.
5. Cool each chaffle completely before serving.

Nutrition

Calories: 162 kcal

Cholesterol: 108 mg

Carbohydrates: 2 g

Protein: 12 g

Fat: 12 g

Sugar: 0 g

Maple Pumpkin Chaffle

Preparation Time: 5 minutes

Cooking Time: 16 minutes

Serving: 2

Ingredients:

- 2 eggs
- 1/2 cup grated mozzarella cheese
- 3/4 tsp. baking powder
- 2 tsp. pureed pumpkin, no additives
- 3/4 tsp. pumpkin pie spice
- 1/2 tsp. vanilla
- pinch of salt
- 4 tsp. heavy whipping cream
- 1 tsp. coconut flour, ALLERGY WARNING

Toppings:

- 2 tsp. sugar-free maple syrup

Directions:

1. Preheat the Chaffle iron.
2. Whisk together all the ingredients well.
3. Add 1/4 of the batter to the Chaffle iron and Cooking for three to four minutes.
4. Repeat until all the batter is finished.

Nutrition

Calories: 201 kcal

Cholesterol: 200 mg

Carbohydrates: 4 g

Protein: 12 g

Fat: 15 g

Sugar: 1 g

Tiramisu Chaffle Cake

Preparation Time: 10 minutes

Cooking Time: 16 minutes

Serving: 4

Ingredients:

Chaffle

- 2 large eggs, room temperature
- 2 tbsp. unsalted butter, melted
- 2 tsp. instant coffee powder
- 1 oz. cream cheese, softened
- 1 tsp. vanilla extract
- 1/4 cup fine almond flour
- 2 tbsp. coconut flour
- 1 tbsp. cocoa powder, gluten-free
- 2 tbsp. powdered sweetener of choice
- 1 tsp. baking powder
- 1/8 tsp. salt

Ingredients For Filling:

- 4 oz. mascarpone cheese
- 1/4 cup powdered sweetener of choice
- 1/2 tsp. vanilla extract

Ingredients for Secondary Filling:

- 1/2 tsp. instant coffee powder
- 1/2 tbsp. cocoa powder, gluten-free

- 1/2 tsp. hazelnut extract, optional

Directions:

Chaffle

1. Preheat the Chaffle iron.
2. Mix the melted butter and the powdered coffee.
3. With this mixture add the extracts, eggs, and cream cheese. Stir well.
4. Add the remaining dry ingredients together and mix well.
5. Pout 1/4 of the mixture into the Chaffle iron and Cooking for about four minutes.
6. Repeat this until all the batter is used.
7. While the fourth chaffle is Cooking, start on the cream filling.

Directions

For the Two Fillings:

1. In a clean bowl mix the mascarpone, vanilla, and sweetener.
2. Divide the filling between two bowls. One will remain white and be the filling between chaffles.
3. Once the chaffles are cool spread the white filling between layers. Refrigerate for about 20 minutes.
4. In the second bowl, add the instant coffee and cocoa and mix well.
5. Take this second filling and coat the stacked chaffles.
6. Refrigerate the cake for another 30 minutes to allow the frosting to set.

Nutrition

Calories: 302 kcal

Carbohydrates: 12 g

Protein: 8 g

Fat: 27 g

Sugar: 6 g

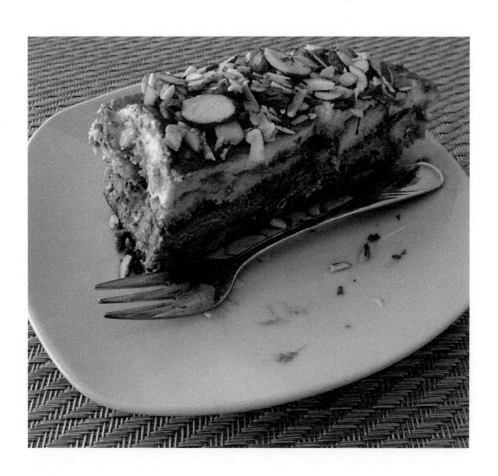

Cinnamon Sugar Chaffle

Preparation Time: 5 minutes

Cooking Time: 8 minutes

Serving: 2

Ingredients:

- 1 large egg
- 1/2 tbsp. melted butter
- 3/4 cup grated mozzarella cheese
- 2 tbsp. almond flour (or 2 tsp. coconut flour),
- 1/2 tsp. vanilla extract
- 2 tbsp. granulated Erythritol, or granulated sweetener of choice
- 1/2 tsp. cinnamon
- 1/2 tsp. psyllium husk powder, optional (for texture)
- 1/4 tsp. baking powder, optional

Topping:

- 3/4 tsp. cinnamon
- 1 tbsp. butter, melted
- 1/4 cup Erythritol, granulated

Directions:

Chaffle

1. Preheat the Chaffle iron.
2. Stir all ingredients together in a bowl. Exclude the topping ingredients.

3. Use half the batter to make one chaffle. Repeat until the batter is finished.
4. Cooking for between three and four minutes or until brown.
5. Remove chaffle from the Chaffle iron and let cool.

Directions

For Toppings:

1. Mix the cinnamon and Erythritol together. This will be used for the topping. Once the chaffles are cooled brush melted butter on the surface. Once covered in melted butter, sprinkle the topping.
2. This delicious treat can be enjoyed with some heavy cream and some berries.

Nutrition

Calories: 179 kcal

Carbohydrates: 2 g net

Protein: 10 g

Fat: 14 g

Sweet Vanilla Chocolate Chaffle

Preparation Time: 5 minutes

Cooking Time: 18 minutes

Serving: 1

Ingredients:

- Egg (1 whisked)
- Vanilla (.5 tsp.)
- Cinnamon (.25 tsp.)
- Swerve (1 tbsp.)
- Unchilled cream cheese (2 oz.)
- Coconut flour (1 tbsp.)
- Unsweetened cocoa powder (2 tsp.)

Directions:

1. Add each of the fixings in a mixing bowl and whisk until incorporated. Heat the Chaffle iron and spritz with a bit of Cooking oil spray.
2. Prepare the chaffle in two batches and Cook them until golden (4- 5 min.).

Nutrition

Calories: 128 kcal

Cholesterol: 104 mg

Carbohydrates: 3 g

Protein: 9.5 g

Fat: 8.7 g

Sugar: 0.7 g

Chocolate Chip Muffins

Preparation Time: 10 minutes

Cooking Time: 20 minutes

Servings: 8

Ingredients

- 1/2 cup coconut flour
- 1/4 tsp. baking soda
- 1/4 tsp. salt
- 4 eggs
- 1/3 cup unsalted butter, melted
- 1/2 cup low-carb sweetener
- 1 Tbsp. vanilla extract
- 2 Tbsp. coconut milk
- 1/3 cup sugar-free chocolate chips

Directions

1. Preheat the oven to 350F.
2. Attach the coconut flour, baking soda, and salt in a bowl and blend well.
3. Add the butter, eggs, sweetener, vanilla, and coconut milk to the dry ingredients and mix well. Gently stir in the chocolate chips.
4. Line muffin tins and fill 3/4.
5. Bake for 20 minutes.
6. Cool and serve.

Nutrition:

Calories: 168

Fat: 13g

Carb: 6g

Protein: 5g

Blueberry Cinnamon Chaffles

Preparation Time: 5 minutes

Cooking Time: 10 minutes

Serving: 3

Ingredients:

1. 1 cup shredded mozzarella cheese
2. 3 Tbsp. almond flour
3. 2 eggs
4. 2 tsp. Swerve or granulated sweetener of choice
5. 1 tsp. cinnamon
6. 1/2 tsp. baking powder
7. 1/2 cup fresh blueberries
8. 1/2 tsp. of powdered Swerve

Directions

1. Turn on Chaffle maker to heat and oil it with Cooking spray.
2. Mix eggs, flour, mozzarella, cinnamon, vanilla extract, sweetener, and baking powder in a bowl until well combined.
3. Add in blueberries.
4. Pour 1/4 batter into each Chaffle mold. Close and Cooking for 8 minutes.
5. If it's crispy and the Chaffle maker opens without pulling the chaffles apart, the chaffle is ready.
6. If not, close and Cooking for 1-2 minutes more.
7. Serve with favorite topping and more blueberries.

Nutrition

Calories: 368 kcal

Carbohydrates: 3 g

Protein: 11 g

Fat: 23 g

Chocolate Chaffles

Preparation Time: 3 minutes

Cooking Time: 10 minutes

Serving: 2

Ingredients:

- 3/4 cup shredded mozzarella
- 1 large egg
- 2 Tbsp. almond flour
- 2 Tbsp. allulose
- 1/2 Tbsp. melted butter
- 11/2 Tbsp. cocoa powder
- 1/2 tsp. vanilla extract
- 1/2 tsp. psyllium husk powder
- 1/4 tsp. baking powder

Directions

1. Turn on Chaffle maker to heat and oil it with Cooking spray.
2. Mix all ingredients in a small bowl.
3. Pour 1/4 cup batter into a 4-inch Chaffle maker.
4. Cooking for 2-3 minutes, or until crispy.
5. Transfer chaffle to a plate and set aside.
6. Repeat with remaining batter.

Nutrition:

Calories 235

Fats 20.62g

Carbs 5.9g

Net Carbs 5g

Protein 7.51g

Raspberry Chaffles

Preparation Time: 5 minutes

Cooking Time: 6 minutes

Serving: 2

Ingredients:

- 4 Tbsp. almond flour
- 4 large eggs
- 2 1/3 cup shredded mozzarella cheese
- 1 tsp. vanilla extract
- 1 Tbsp. Erythritol sweetener
- 11/2 tsp. baking powder
- 1/2 cup raspberries

Directions

1. Turn on Chaffle maker to heat and oil it with Cooking spray.
2. Mix almond flour, sweetener, and baking powder in a bowl.
3. Add cheese, eggs, and vanilla extract, and mix until well-combined.
4. Add 1 portion of batter to Chaffle maker and spread it evenly.
5. Close and Cooking for 3-4 minutes, or until golden.
6. Repeat until remaining batter is used.
7. Serve with raspberries.

Nutrition

Calories: 162 kcal

Cholesterol: 108 mg

Carbohydrates: 2 g

Protein: 12 g

Strawberry Shortcake Chaffles

Preparation Time: 20 minutes

Cooking Time: 25 minutes

Serving: 1

Ingredients:

For the batter:

- 1 egg
- 1/4 cup mozzarella cheese
- 1 Tbsp. cream cheese
- 1/4 tsp. baking powder
- 2 strawberries, sliced
- 1 tsp. strawberry extract

For the glaze:

- 1 Tbsp. cream cheese
- 1/4 tsp. strawberry extract
- 1 Tbsp. monk fruit confectioners blend

For the whipped cream:

- 1 cup heavy whipping cream
- 1 tsp. vanilla
- 1 Tbsp. monk fruit

Directions

1. Turn on Chaffle maker to heat and oil it with Cooking spray.
2. Beat egg in a small bowl.
3. Add remaining batter components.

4. Divide the mixture in half.

5. Cooking one half of the batter in a Chaffle maker for 4 minutes, or until golden brown. Repeat with remaining batter

6. Mix all glaze ingredients and spread over each warm chaffle.

7. Mix all whipped cream ingredients and whip until it starts to form peaks.

8. Top each Chaffle with whipped cream and strawberries.

Nutrition

Calories: 119 kcal

Cholesterol: 111 mg

Carbohydrates: 2.7 g

Protein: 8.8 g

Glazed Chaffles

Preparation Time: 10 minutes

Cooking Time: 5 minutes

Serving: 2

Ingredients:

- 1/2 cup mozzarella shredded cheese
- 1/8 cup cream cheese
- 2 Tbsp. unflavored whey protein isolate
- 2 Tbsp. swerve confectioners' sugar substitute
- 1/2 tsp. baking powder
- 1/2 tsp. vanilla extract
- 1 egg

For the glaze topping:

- 2 Tbsp. heavy whipping cream
- 3-4 Tbsp. swerve confectioners' sugar substitute
- 1/2 tsp. vanilla extract

Directions

1. Turn on Chaffle maker to heat and oil it with Cooking spray.
2. In a microwave-safe bowl, mix mozzarella and cream cheese. Set at 30 second intervals until melted and fully combined.
3. Add protein, 2 Tbsp. sweetener, baking powder to cheese. Knead with hands until well incorporated.
4. Place dough into a mixing bowl and beat in egg and vanilla until a smooth batter forms.

5. Put 1/3 of the batter into Chaffle maker, and Cooking for 3-5 minutes, until golden brown.
6. Repeat until all 3 chaffles are made.
7. Beat glaze ingredients in a bowl and pour over chaffles before serving.

Nutrition:

Cal 215

Net Carbs 4g

Fat 15g

Protein 12g

Lemon Curd Chaffles

Preparation Time: 40 minutes

Cooking Time: 5 minutes

Serving: 1

Ingredients:

- 3 large eggs
- 4 oz. cream cheese, softened
- 1 Tbsp. low carb sweetener
- 1 tsp. vanilla extract
- 3/4 cup mozzarella cheese, shredded
- 3 Tbsp. coconut flour
- 1 tsp. baking powder
- 1/3 tsp. salt

For the lemon curd:

- 1/2-1 cup water
- 5 egg yolks
- 1/2 cup lemon juice
- 1/2 cup powdered sweetener
- 2 Tbsp. fresh lemon zest
- 1 tsp. vanilla extract Pinch of salt
- 8 Tbsp. cold butter, cubed

Directions

1. Pour water into a saucepan and heat over medium until it reaches a soft boil. Start with 1/2 cup and add more if needed.
2. Whisk yolks, lemon juice, lemon zest, powdered sweetener, vanilla, and salt in a medium heat-proof bowl. Leave to set for 5-6 minutes.
3. Place bowl onto saucepan and heat. The bowl shouldn't be touching water.
4. Whisk mixture for 8-10 minutes, or until it begins to thicken.
5. Add butter cubes and whisk for 5-7 minutes, until it thickens. When it lightly coats the back of a spoon, remove from heat.
6. Refrigerate until cool, allowing it to continue thickening.
7. Turn on Chaffle maker to heat and oil it with Cooking spray.
8. Add baking powder, coconut flour, and salt in a small bowl. Mix well and set aside.
9. Add eggs, cream cheese, sweetener, and vanilla in a separate bowl. Using a hand beater, beat until frothy.
10. Add mozzarella to egg mixture and beat again.
11. Add dry ingredients and mix until well-combined.
12. Add batter to Chaffle maker and Cooking for 3-4 minutes.
13. Transfer to a plate and top with lemon curd before serving.

Nutrition:

Cal 263

Net Carbs: 6g

Fat: 22g

Protein: 10g

Chaffle Churros

Preparation Time: 10 minutes

Cooking Time: 6 minutes

Serving: 2

Ingredients:

- 1 egg
- 1 Tbsp. almond flour
- 1/2 tsp. vanilla extract
- 1 tsp. cinnamon, divided
- 1/4 tsp. baking powder
- 1/2 cup shredded mozzarella
- 1 Tbsp. swerve confectioners' sugar substitute
- 1 Tbsp. swerve brown sugar substitute
- 1 Tbsp. butter, melted

Directions

1. Turn on Chaffle maker to heat and oil it with Cooking spray.
2. Mix egg, flour, vanilla extract, 1/2 tsp. cinnamon, baking powder, mozzarella, and sugar substitute in a bowl.
3. Place half of the mixture into Chaffle maker and Cooking for 3-5 minutes, or until desired doneness.
4. Remove and place the second half of the batter into the maker.
5. Cut chaffles into strips.
6. Place strips in a bowl and cover with melted butter.

7. Mix brown sugar substitute and the remaining cinnamon in a bowl.
8. Pour sugar mixture over the strips and toss to coat them well.

Nutrition:

Calories: 77

Net Carb: 2.4g

Fat: 9.8g

Carbohydrates: 3.2g

Dietary Fiber: 0.8g

Blueberry Chaffles

Preparation Time: 5 minutes

Cooking Time: 15 minutes

Serving: 4

Ingredients:

- 2 eggs
- 1/2 cup blueberries
- 1/2 tsp. baking powder
- 1/2 tsp. vanilla
- 2 tsp. Swerve
- 3 tbsp. almond flour
- 1 cup mozzarella cheese, shredded

Directions:

1. Preheat your Chaffle maker.
2. In a medium bowl, mix eggs, vanilla, Swerve, almond flour, and cheese.
3. Add blueberries and stir well.
4. Spray Chaffle maker with Cooking spray.
5. Pour 1/4 batter in the hot Chaffle maker and Cooking for 8 minutes or until golden brown. Repeat with the remaining batter.
6. Serve and enjoy.

Nutrition:

Cal 89

Net Carbs 5.9g

Fat 6g

Protein 2g

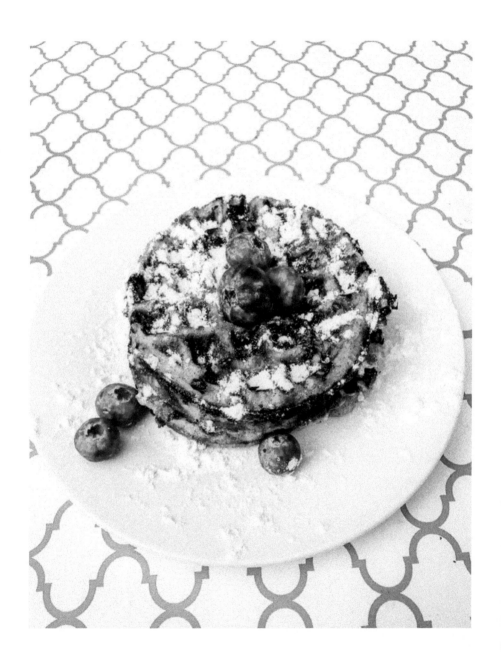

Chaffles with Caramelized Apples And Yogurt

Preparation Time: 5 minutes

Cooking Time: 11 minutes

Serving: 2

Ingredients:

- 1 tablespoon unsalted butter
- 1 tablespoon golden brown sugar
- 1 Granny Smith apple
- 1 pinch salt
- 2 whole-grain frozen Chaffles, toasted
- 1/2 cup mozzarella cheese, shredded
- 1/4 cup Original French Vanilla yogurt

Directions:

1. Dissolved the butter in a large skillet over medium-high heat until starting to brown.
2. Add mozzarella cheese and stir well.
3. Add the sugar, apple slices and salt and Cooking, stirring frequently, until apples are softened and tender, about 6 to 9 minutes.
4. Put one warm Chaffle each on a plate, top each with yogurt and apples.
5. Serve warm.

Nutrition:

Cal 467

Net Carbs 3.2g;

Fat 37g

Protein 27g

Chocolate Brownie Chaffles

Preparation Time: 5 minutes

Cooking Time: 5 minutes

Serving: 2

Ingredients:

- 2 tbsp. cocoa powder
- 1 egg
- 1/4 tsp. baking powder
- 1 tbsp. heavy whipping cream
- 1/2 cup mozzarella cheese

Directions:

1. Set egg with a fork in a small mixing bowl.
2. Add the remaining ingredients in a beaten egg and beat well with a beater until the mixture is smooth and fluffy.
3. Pour batter in a greased preheated Chaffle maker.
4. Close the lid.
5. Cooking chaffles for about 4 minutes until they are thoroughly cooked.
6. Serve with berries and enjoy!

Nutrition:

Calories: 264

Net Carb: 1.7g

Fat: 20g

Carbohydrates: 2.1g

Keto-Peanut Butter Chaffle

Preparation Time: 5 minutes

Cooking Time: 5 minutes

Serving: 2

Ingredients:

- 1 egg
- 1 Tbsp. heavy cream
- 1 Tbsp. unsweetened cocoa
- 1 Tbsp. lakanto powdered sweetener
- 1 tsp. coconut flour
- 1/2 tsp. vanilla extract
- 1/2 tsp. cake batter flavor
- 1/4 tsp. baking powder
- For the filling:
- 3 Tbsp. all-natural peanut butter
- 2 tsp. lakanto powdered sweetener
- 2 Tbsp. heavy cream

Directions

1. Turn on Chaffle maker to heat and oil it with Cooking spray.
2. Mix all chaffle components in a small bowl.
3. Pour half of the mixture into Chaffle maker.
4. Cooking for 3-5 minutes. Remove and repeat for remaining batter.
5. Allow chaffles to sit for 4-5 minutes so that they crisp up.

6. Mix filling ingredients together and spread it between chaffles.

Nutrition:

Calories: 122

Net Carb: 0.5g

Fat: 9.4g

Carbohydrates: 0.5g